ZOOFLIPZ

C0-BLE-923

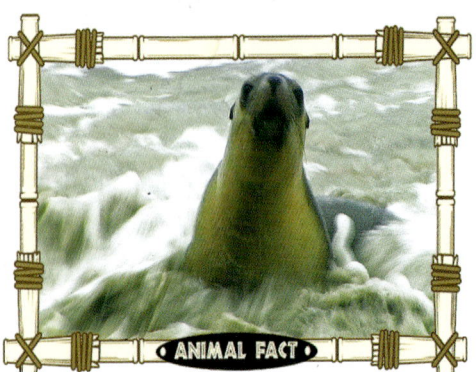

ANIMAL FACT

CREDITS: Sequences—(underwater)©Skip Stubbs/
FOOTAGE SEARCH; (surf) Thought Equity Motion.
Photos—Front, back covers: Reinhard Dirscherl/
Ocean-Photo. Inside covers: Michael Baird

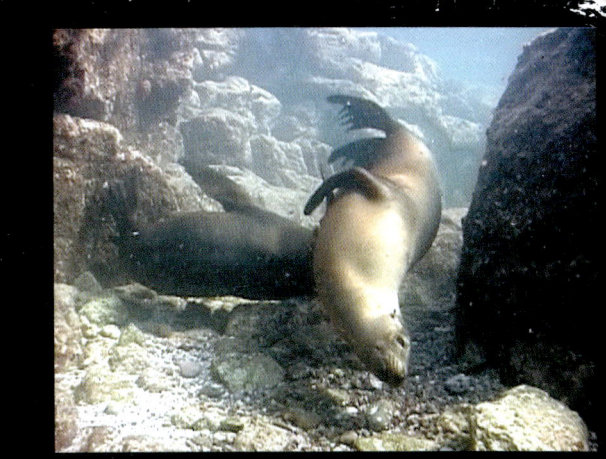

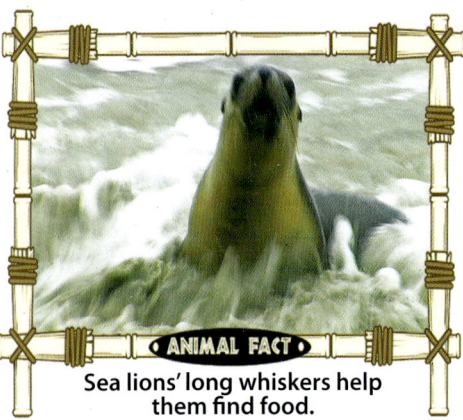

ANIMAL FACT

Sea lions' long whiskers help
them find food.

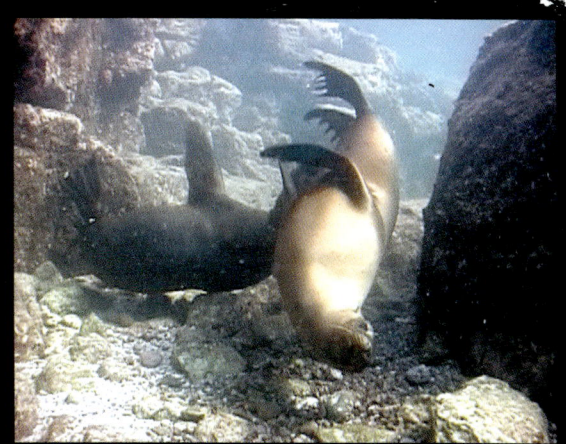

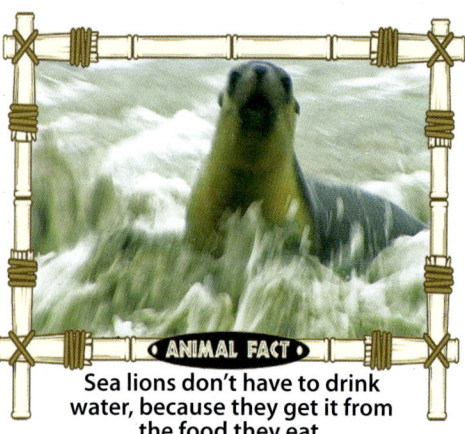

• ANIMAL FACT •

Sea lions don't have to drink
water, because they get it from
the food they eat.

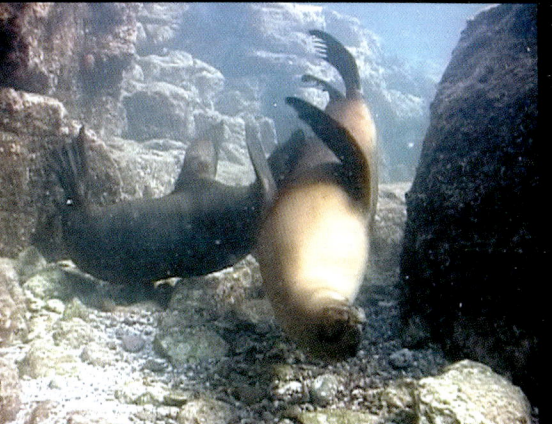

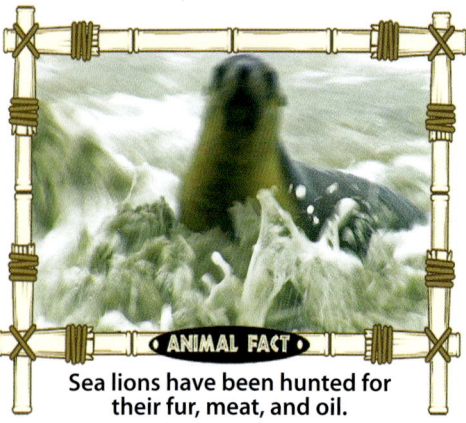

ANIMAL FACT

Sea lions have been hunted for
their fur, meat, and oil.

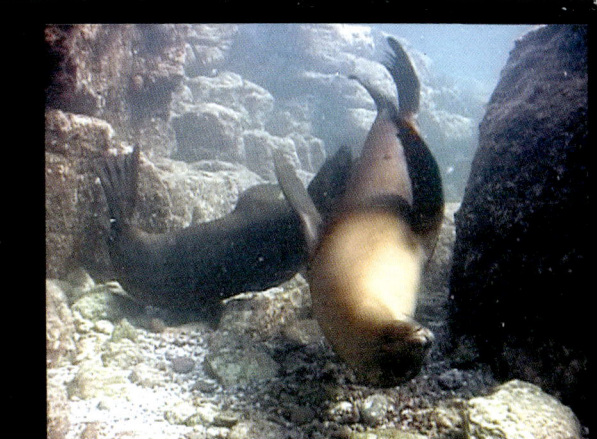

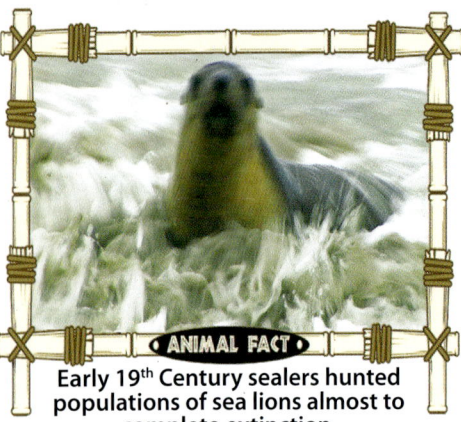

ANIMAL FACT

Early 19th Century sealers hunted populations of sea lions almost to complete extinction.

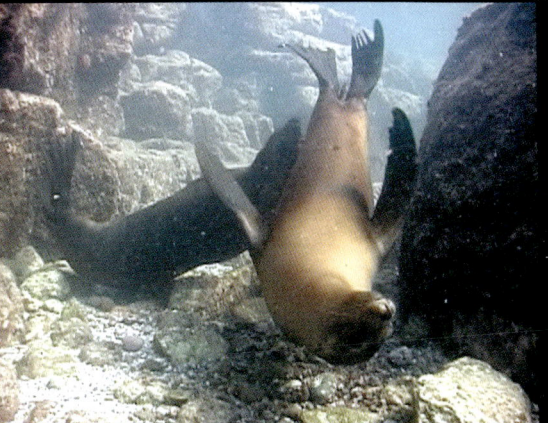

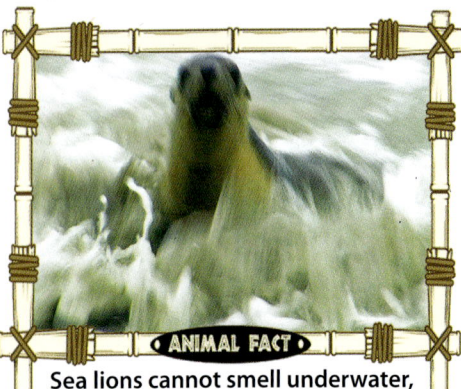

ANIMAL FACT

Sea lions cannot smell underwater,
but have keen noses on land.

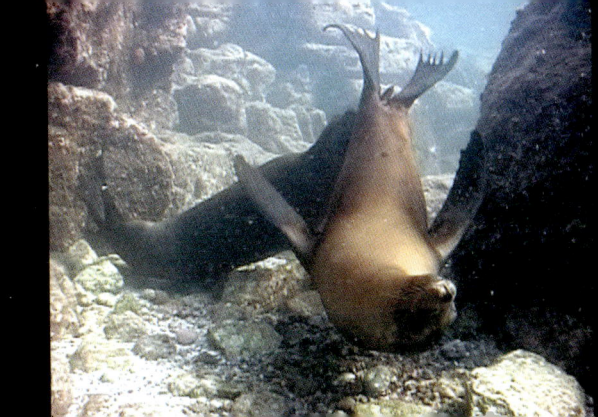

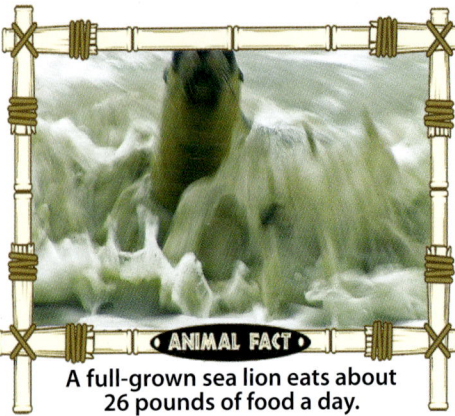

ANIMAL FACT

A full-grown sea lion eats about
26 pounds of food a day.

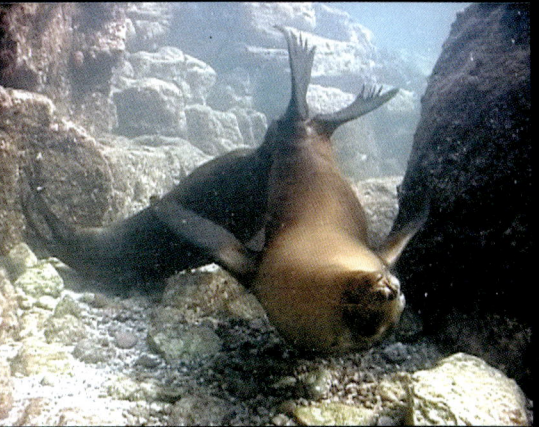

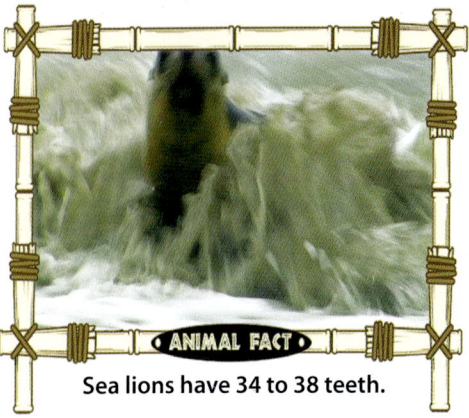

ANIMAL FACT

Sea lions have 34 to 38 teeth.

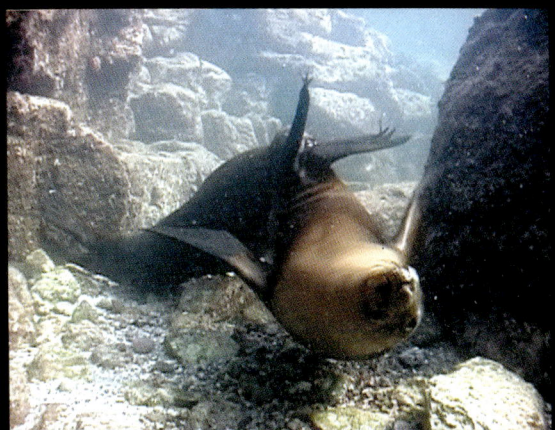

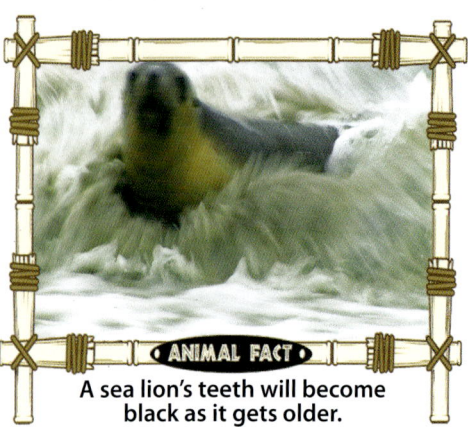

ANIMAL FACT

A sea lion's teeth will become
black as it gets older.

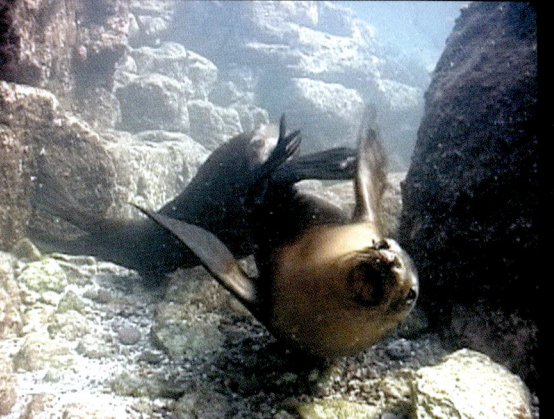

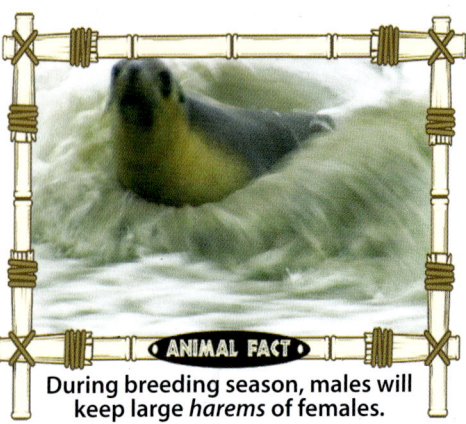

ANIMAL FACT

During breeding season, males will keep large *harems* of females.

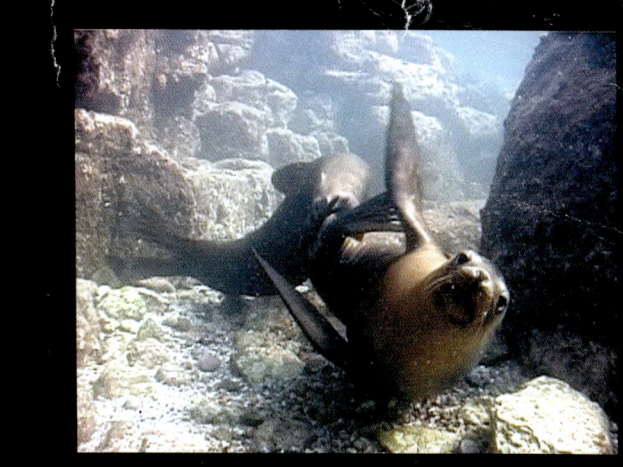

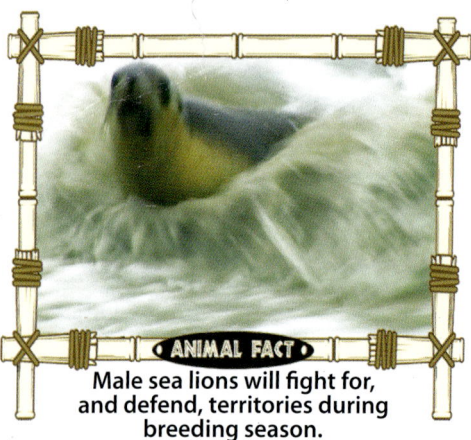

ANIMAL FACT

Male sea lions will fight for,
and defend, territories during
breeding season.

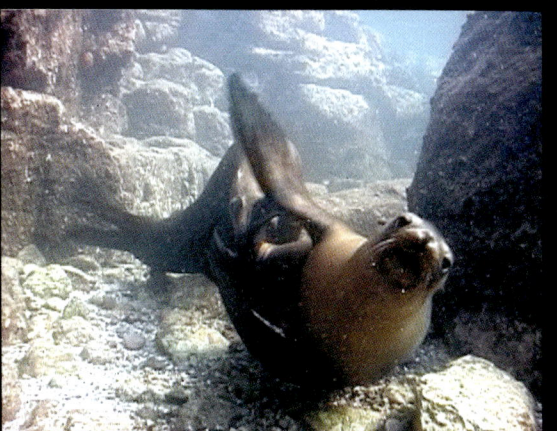

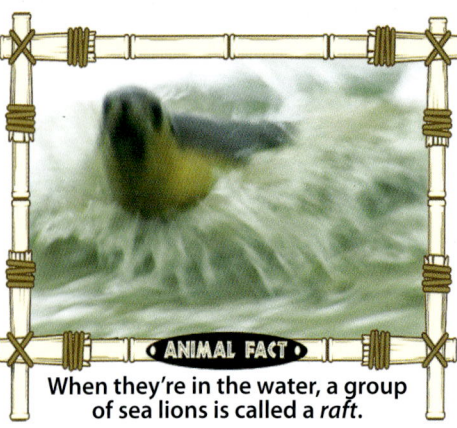

ANIMAL FACT

When they're in the water, a group
of sea lions is called a *raft*.

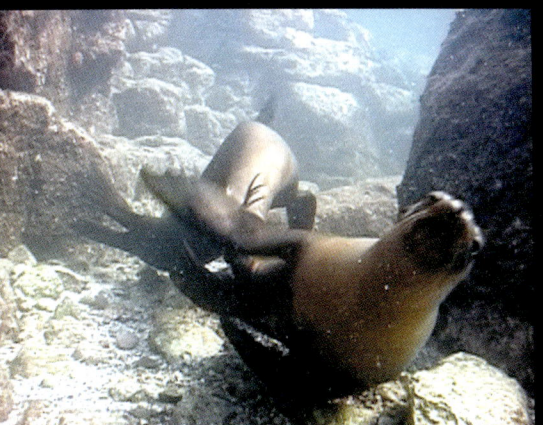

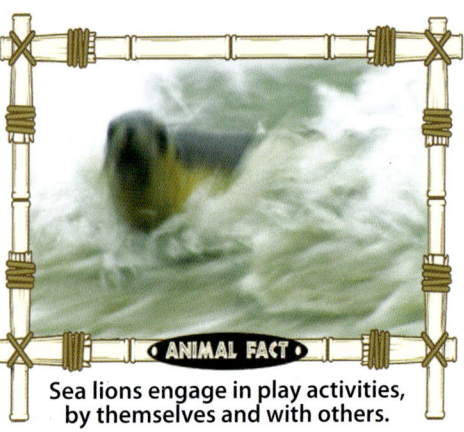

ANIMAL FACT

Sea lions engage in play activities,
by themselves and with others.

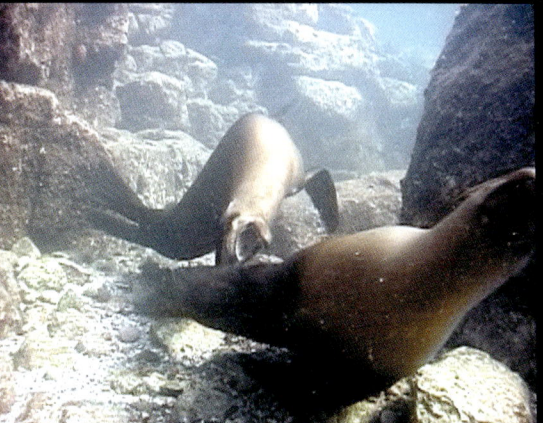

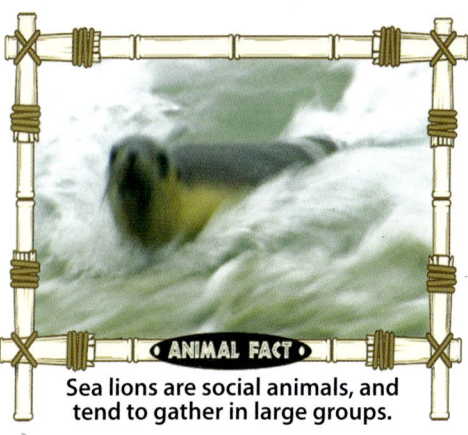

ANIMAL FACT

Sea lions are social animals, and
tend to gather in large groups.

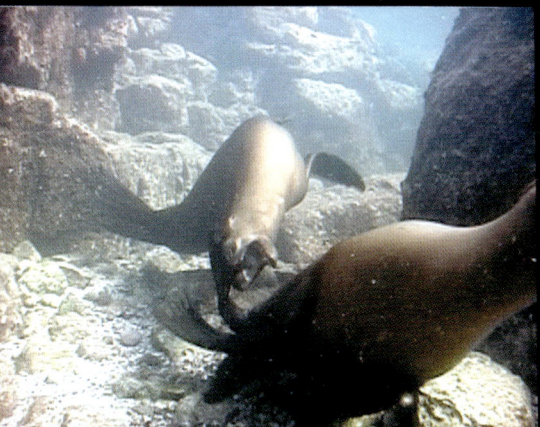

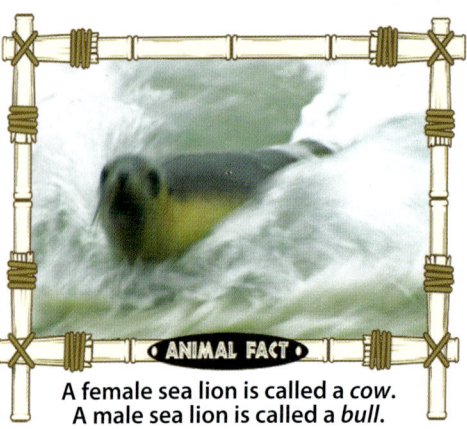

ANIMAL FACT

A female sea lion is called a *cow*.
A male sea lion is called a *bull*.

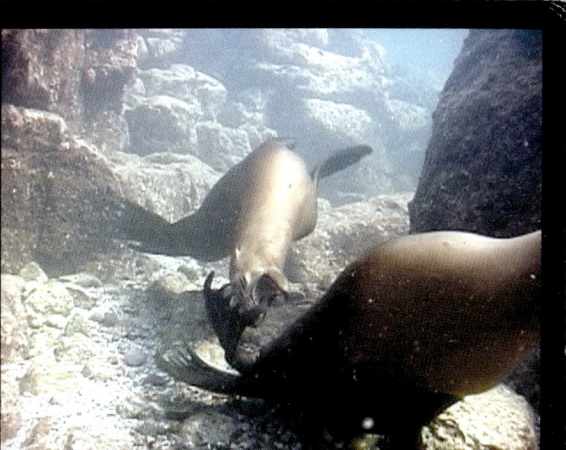

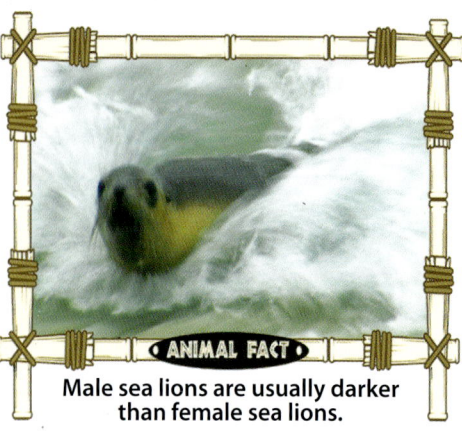

ANIMAL FACT

Male sea lions are usually darker
than female sea lions.

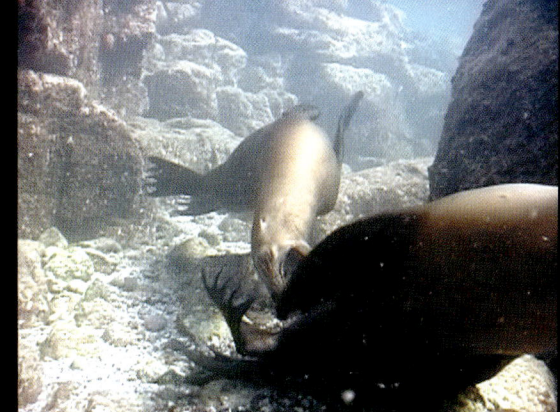

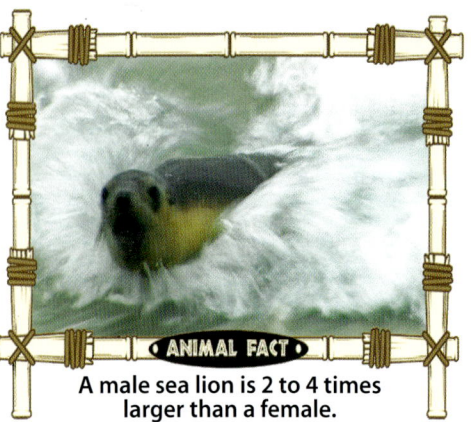

ANIMAL FACT

A male sea lion is 2 to 4 times
larger than a female.

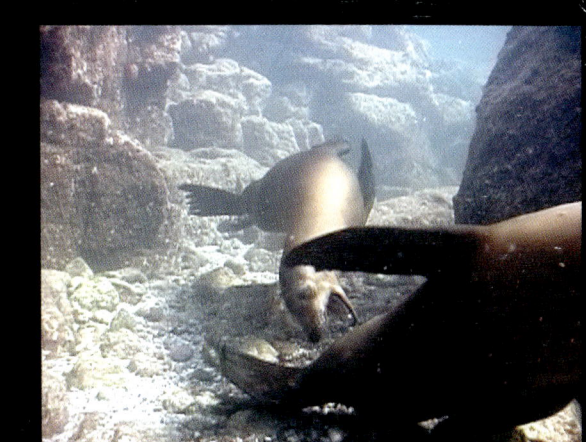

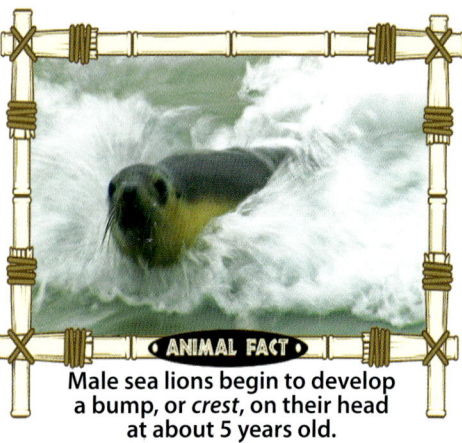

ANIMAL FACT

Male sea lions begin to develop
a bump, or *crest*, on their head
at about 5 years old.

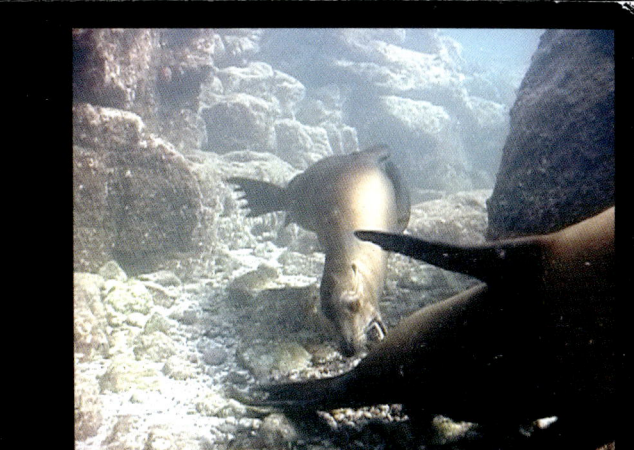

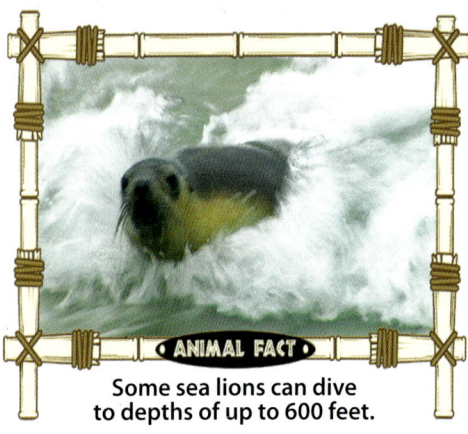

◄ ANIMAL FACT ►

Some sea lions can dive
to depths of up to 600 feet.

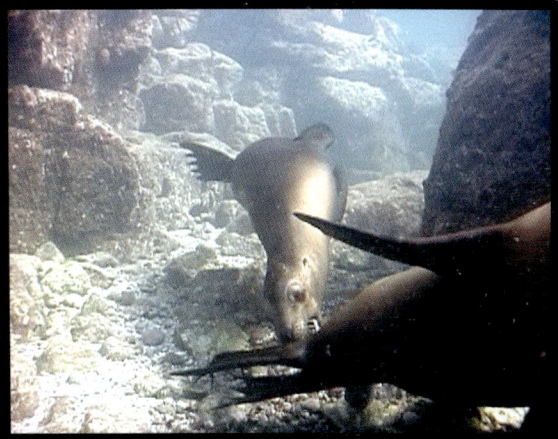

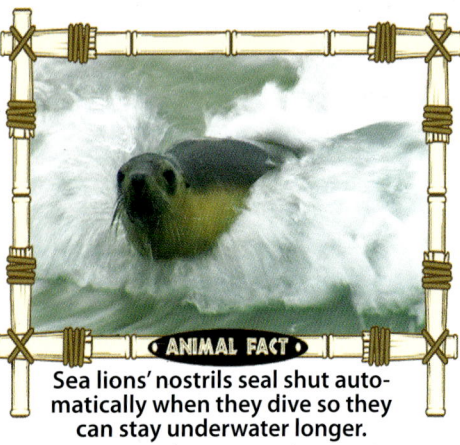

ANIMAL FACT

Sea lions' nostrils seal shut auto-
matically when they dive so they
can stay underwater longer.

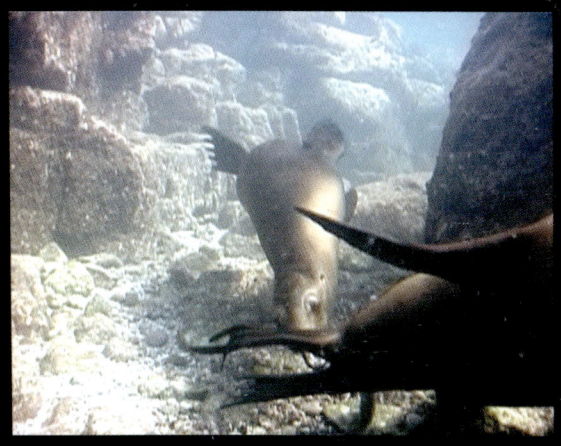

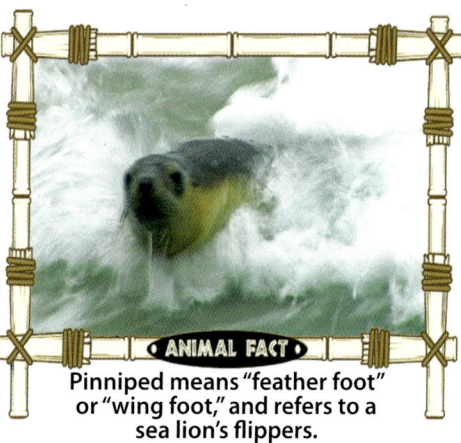

ANIMAL FACT

Pinniped means "feather foot"
or "wing foot," and refers to a
sea lion's flippers.

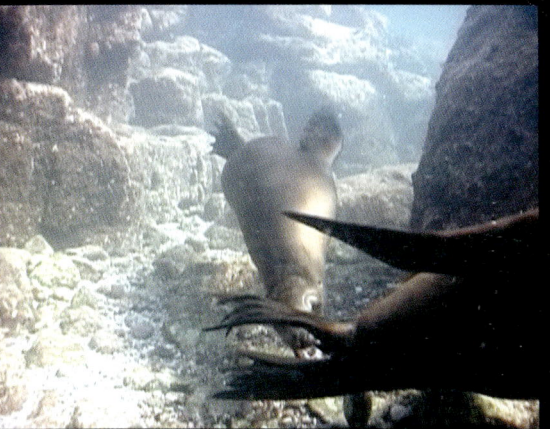

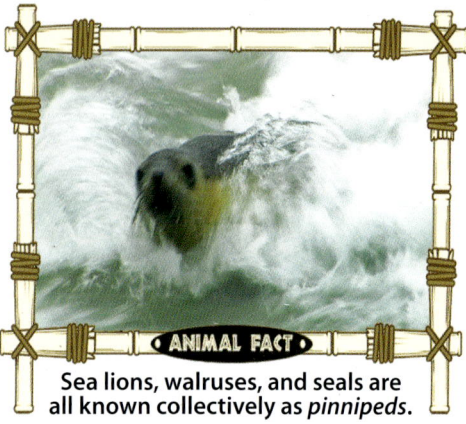

ANIMAL FACT

Sea lions, walruses, and seals are
all known collectively as *pinnipeds*.

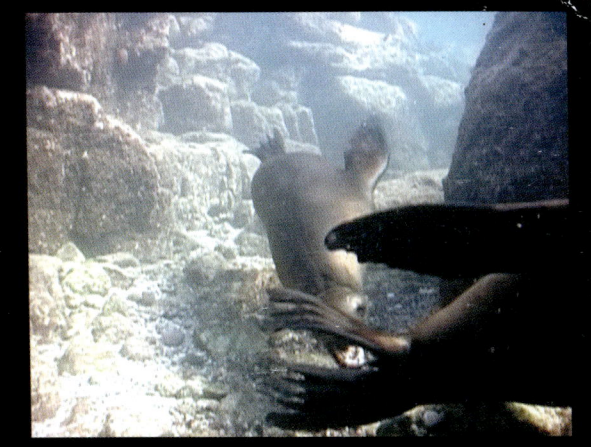

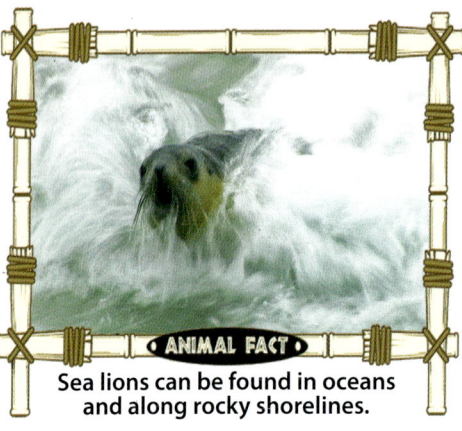

ANIMAL FACT

Sea lions can be found in oceans
and along rocky shorelines.

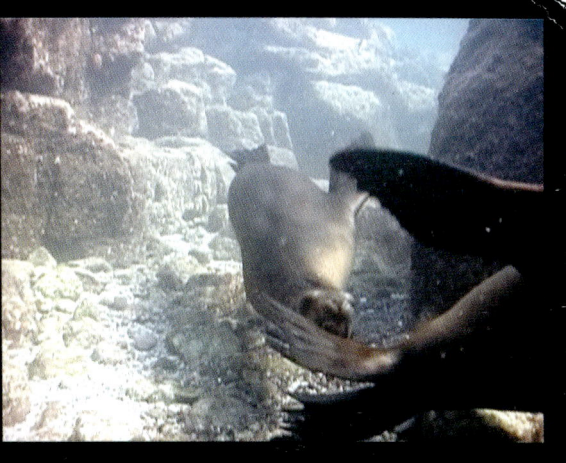

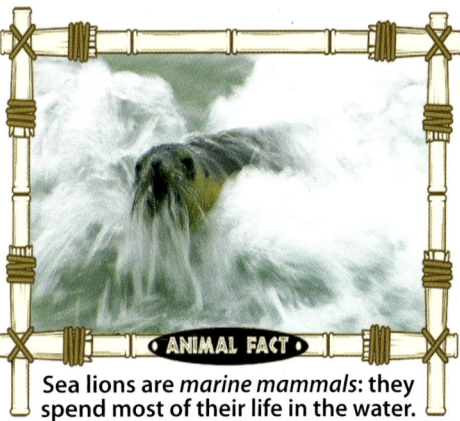

ANIMAL FACT

Sea lions are *marine mammals*: they spend most of their life in the water.

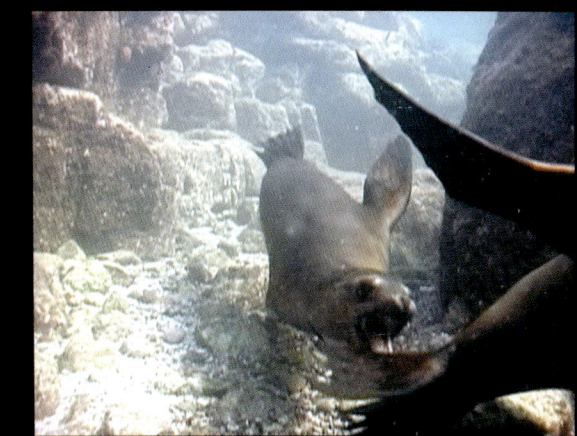

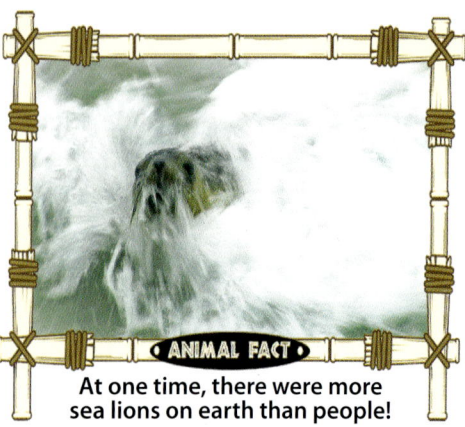

ANIMAL FACT

At one time, there were more
sea lions on earth than people!

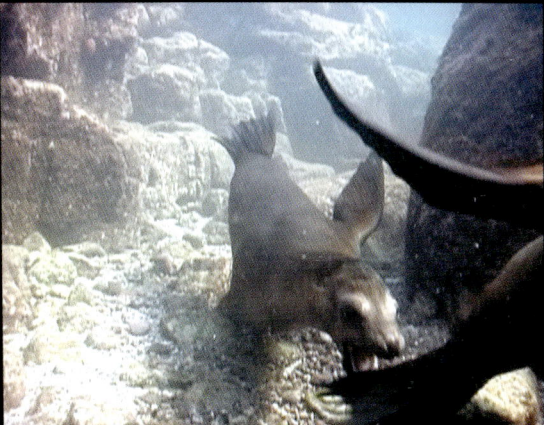

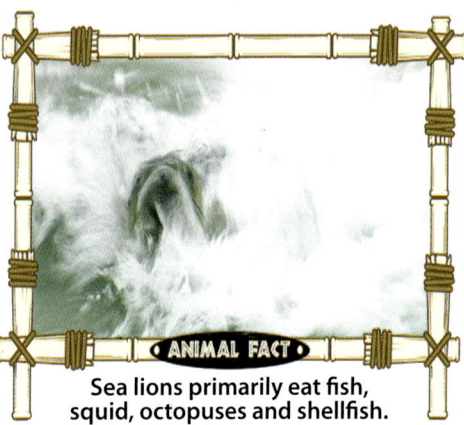

ANIMAL FACT

Sea lions primarily eat fish,
squid, octopuses and shellfish.

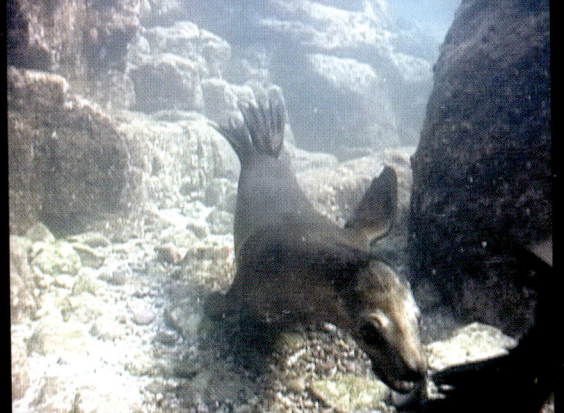

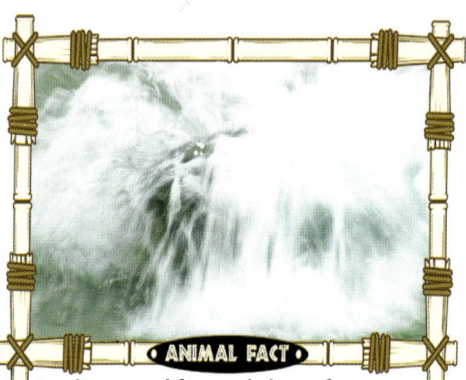

ANIMAL FACT

Sea lions and fur seals have furry *ear-flaps*, which true seals do not have.

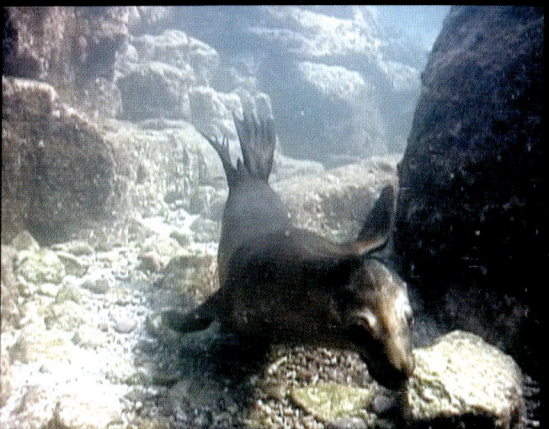

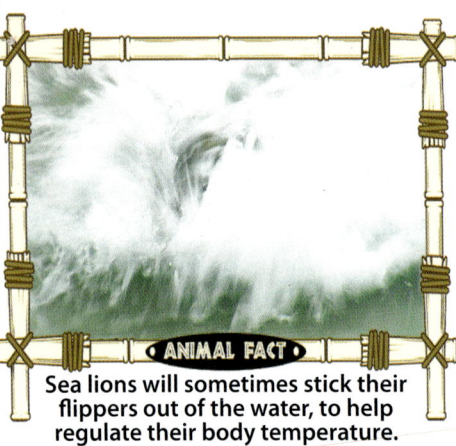

ANIMAL FACT

Sea lions will sometimes stick their
flippers out of the water, to help
regulate their body temperature.

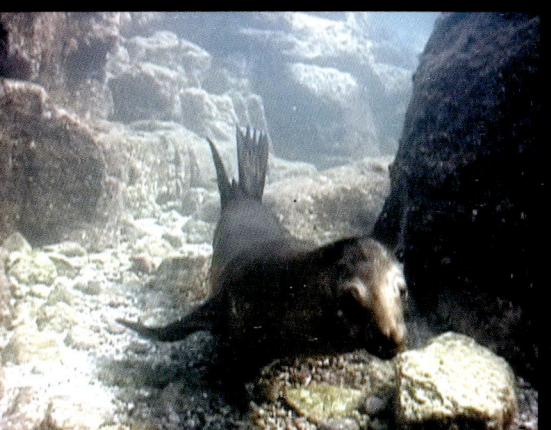

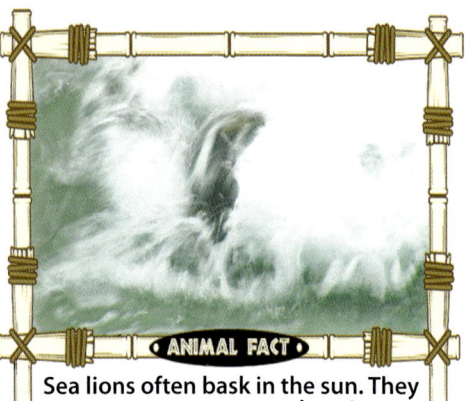

ANIMAL FACT

Sea lions often bask in the sun. They can even get a sunburn!

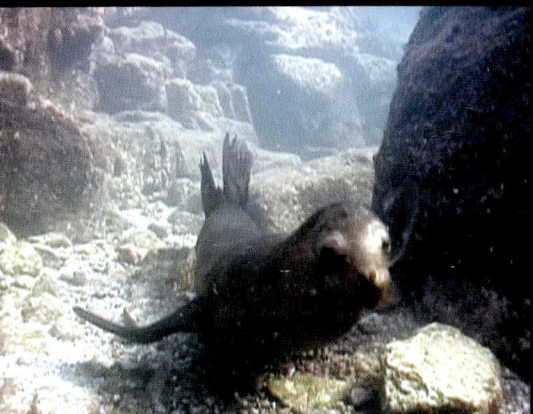

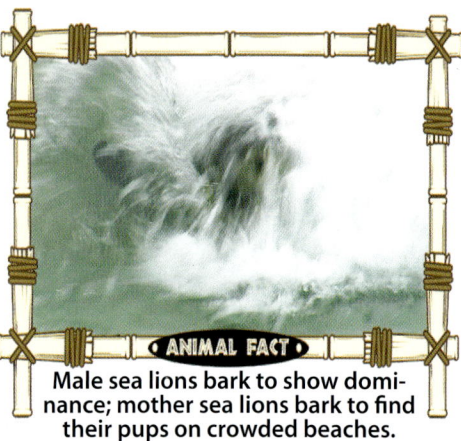

Male sea lions bark to show dominance; mother sea lions bark to find
their pups on crowded beaches.

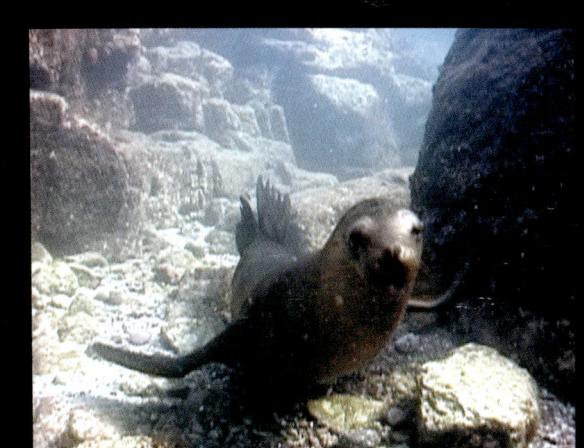

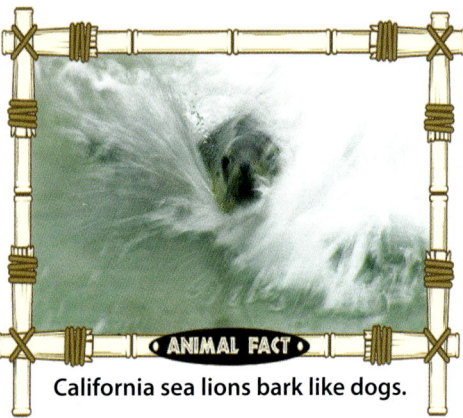

ANIMAL FACT

California sea lions bark like dogs.

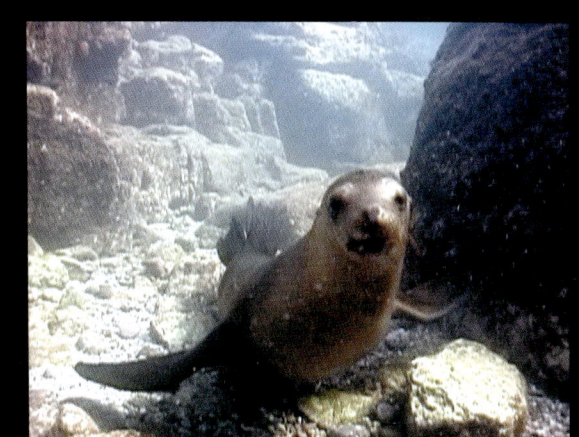

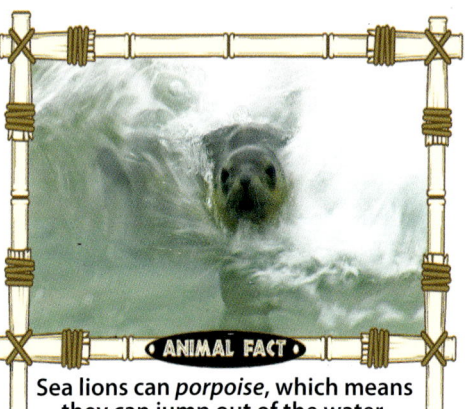

● ANIMAL FACT ●

Sea lions can *porpoise*, which means
they can jump out of the water.

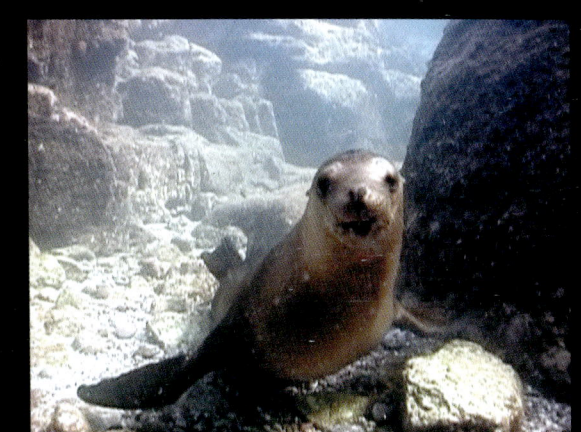

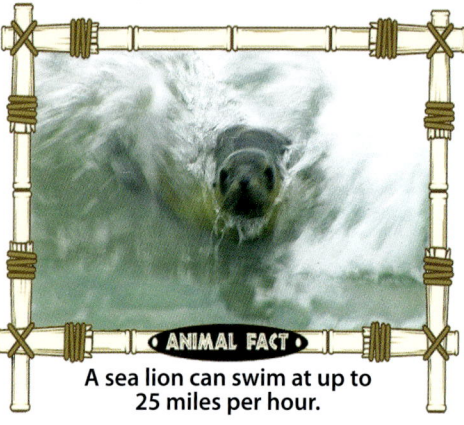

• ANIMAL FACT •

A sea lion can swim at up to
25 miles per hour.

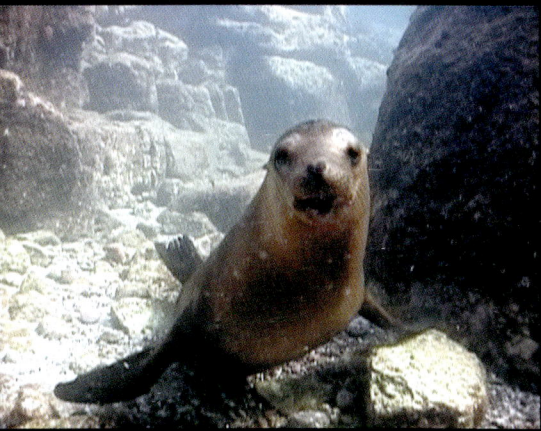

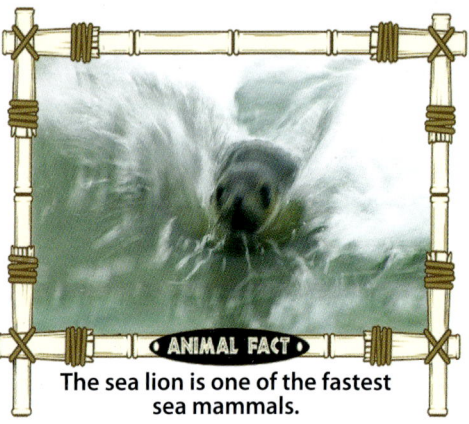

ANIMAL FACT

The sea lion is one of the fastest
sea mammals.

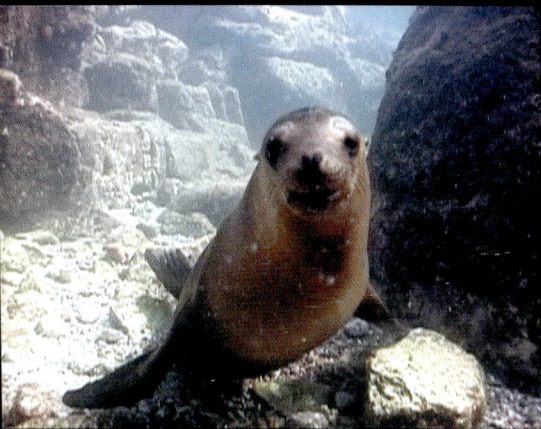

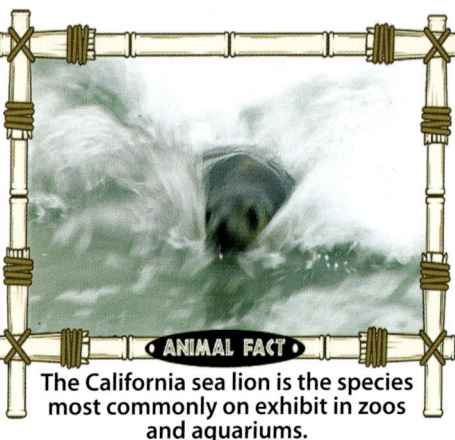

ANIMAL FACT

The California sea lion is the species
most commonly on exhibit in zoos
and aquariums.

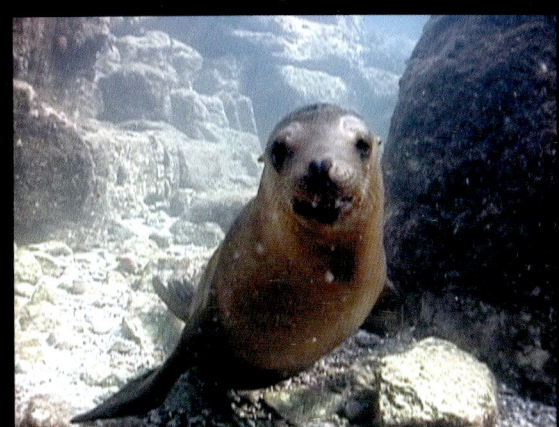

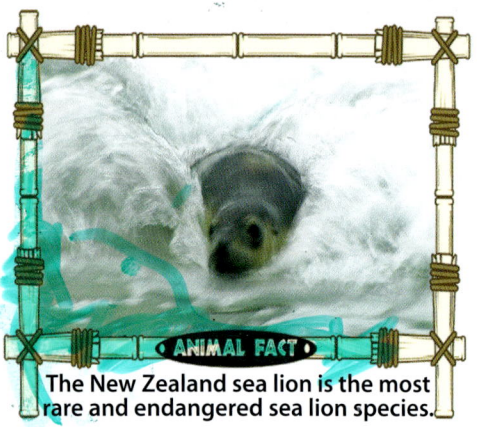

ANIMAL FACT

The New Zealand sea lion is the most
rare and endangered sea lion species.

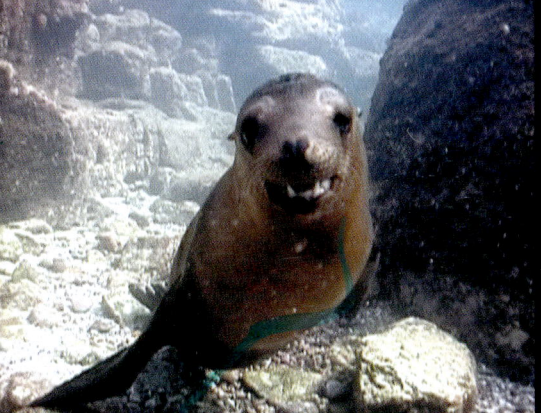

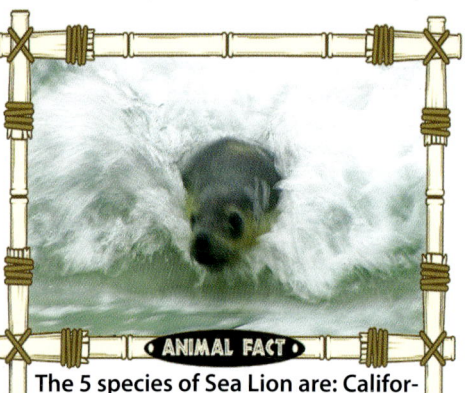

ANIMAL FACT

The 5 species of Sea Lion are: California, Steller, Galapagos or South American, Australian, and New Zealand.

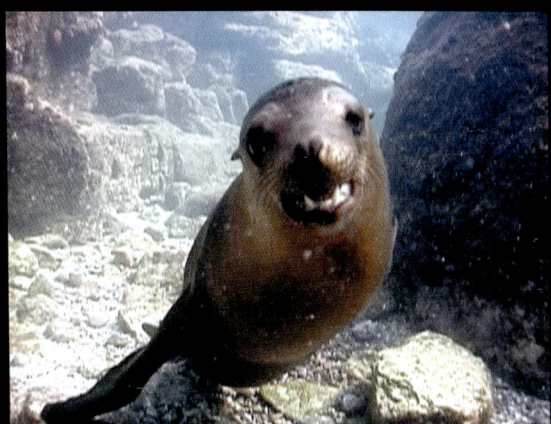

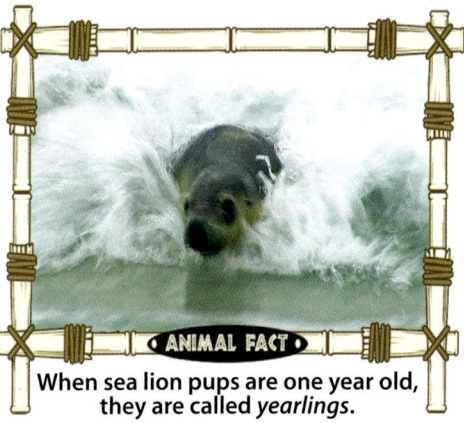

ANIMAL FACT

When sea lion pups are one year old,
they are called *yearlings*.

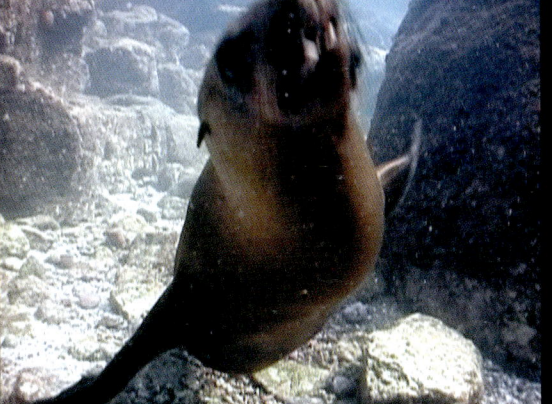

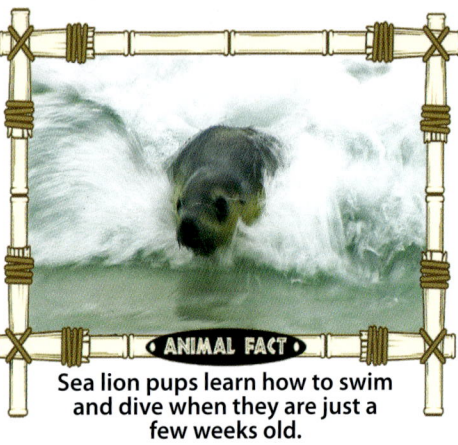

ANIMAL FACT

Sea lion pups learn how to swim
and dive when they are just a
few weeks old.

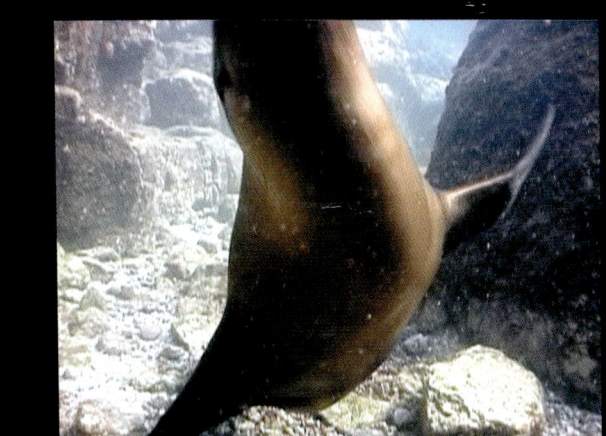

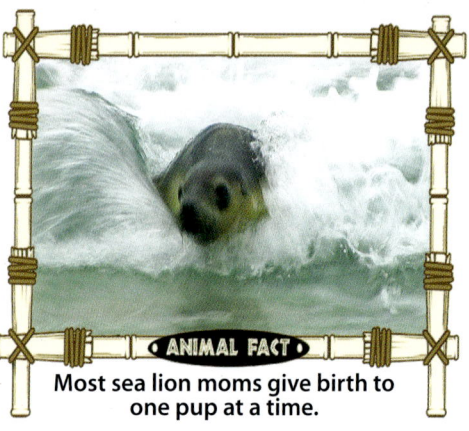

ANIMAL FACT

Most sea lion moms give birth to
one pup at a time.

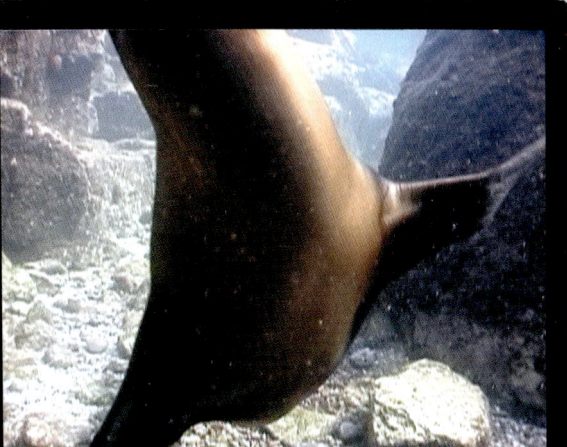

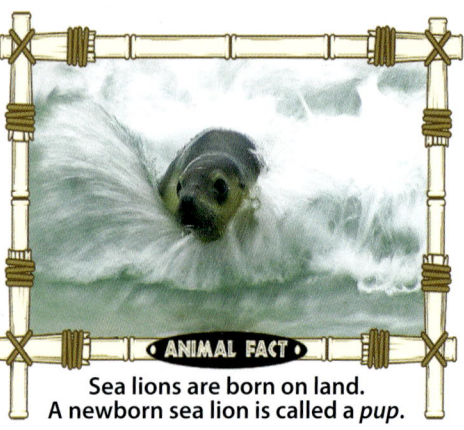

ANIMAL FACT

Sea lions are born on land.
A newborn sea lion is called a *pup*.

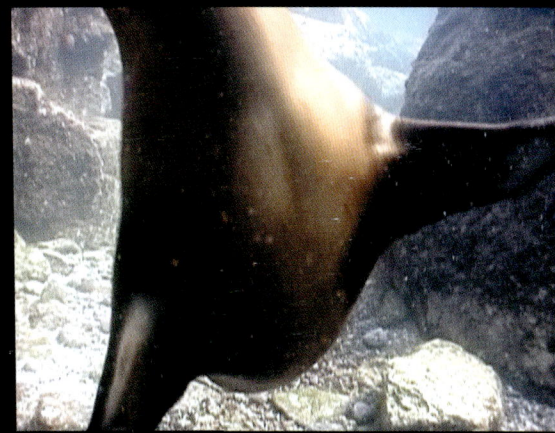

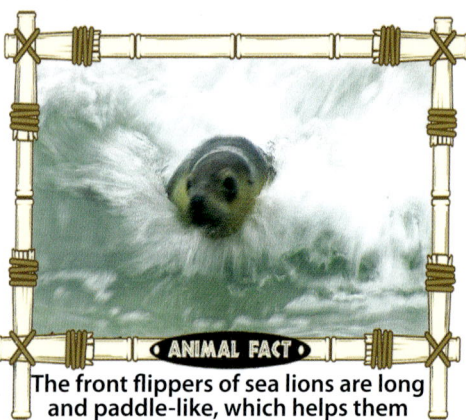

ANIMAL FACT

The front flippers of sea lions are long
and paddle-like, which helps them
get around when they're on land.

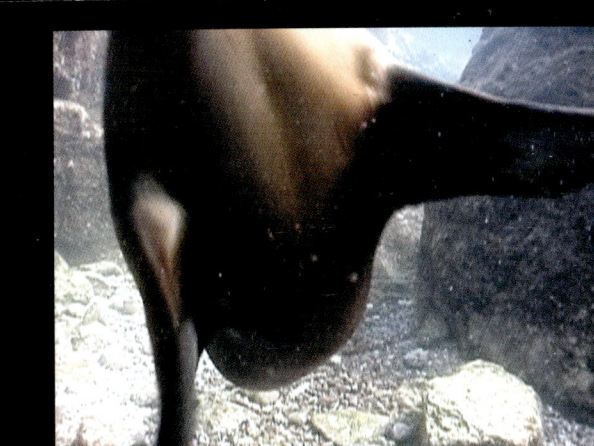

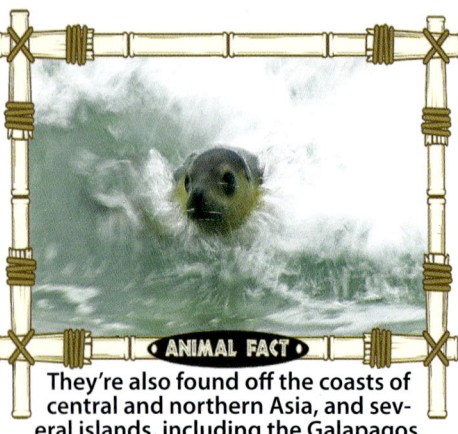

ANIMAL FACT

They're also found off the coasts of central and northern Asia, and several islands, including the Galapagos.

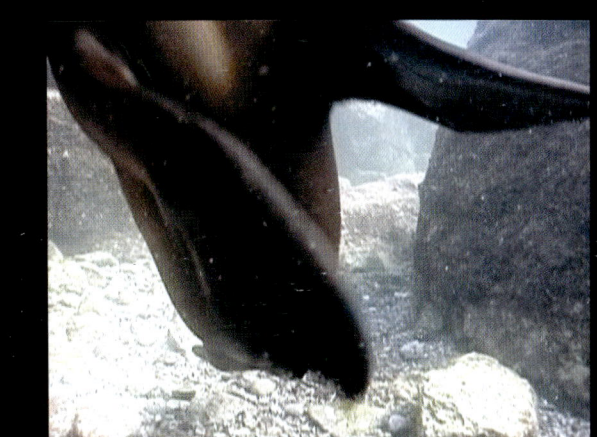

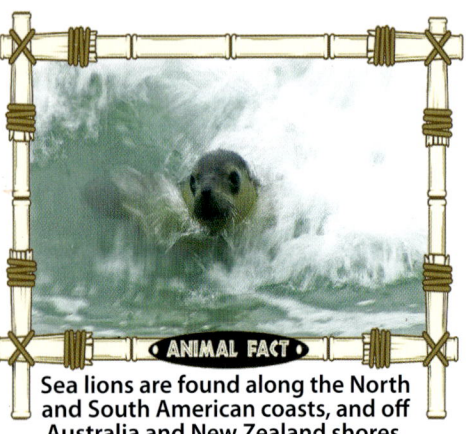

ANIMAL FACT

Sea lions are found along the North and South American coasts, and off Australia and New Zealand shores.

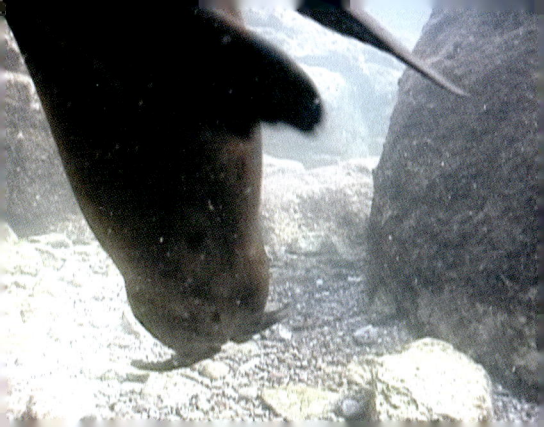

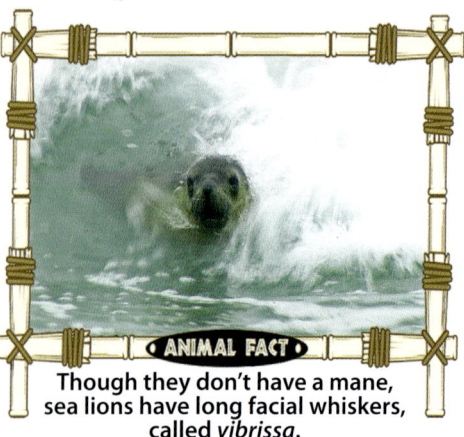

◄ ANIMAL FACT ►

Though they don't have a mane,
sea lions have long facial whiskers,
called *vibrissa*.

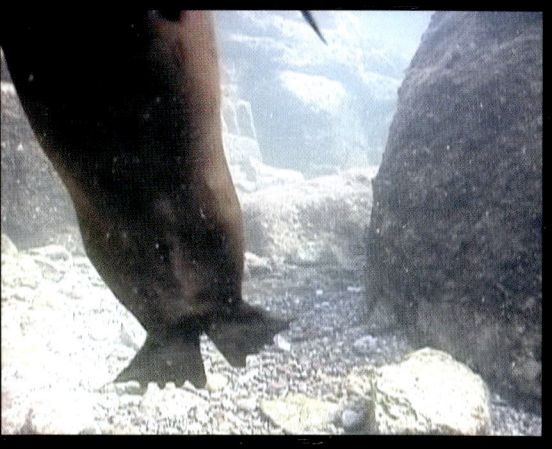

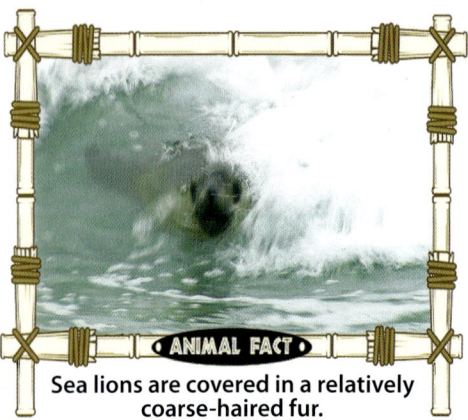

ANIMAL FACT

Sea lions are covered in a relatively
coarse-haired fur.

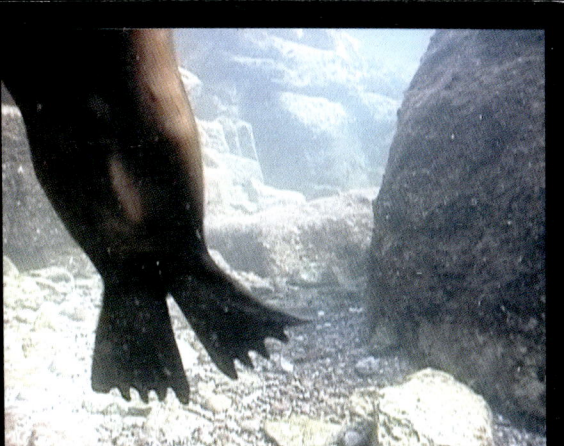

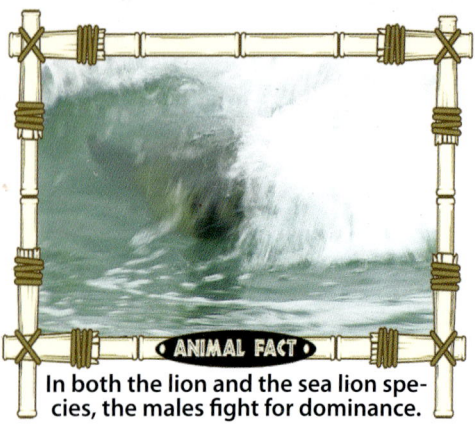

◄ ANIMAL FACT ►

In both the lion and the sea lion species, the males fight for dominance.

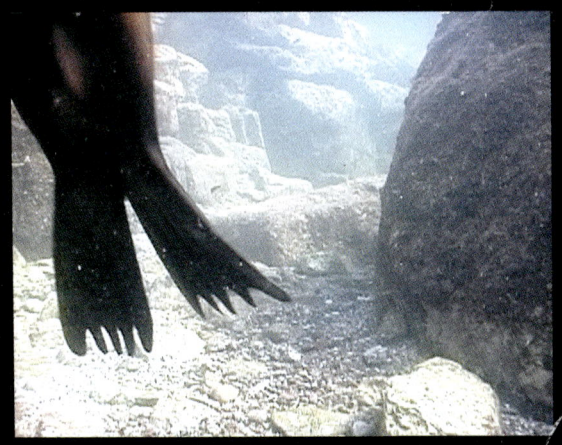

ZOOFLIPZ®

• ANIMAL FACT •

Sea lions are named after the
lions that live on land.